Making Time for Patients:

A Handbook for Ward Sisters

LONDON: HMSO

© Crown copyright 1992
Applications for reproduction should be made to HMSO
First published in August 1992
Second impression November 1992
Third impression April 1993
Printed in the UK for the Audit Commission at Potten Baber & Murray
ISBN 011 886 0879

London : HMSO

Audit Commission, National Health Service Handbook

Table of Contents

1

Introduction

1. The purpose of this handbook on hospital nursing is to help ward-based nurses and the managers closest to the wards improve the quality of patient care in NHS hospitals. It is called 'Making Time for Patients' because, so often, nurses and their managers identify their own lack of time as the **principal** obstacle in the way of making the changes they want to make and that they feel will improve quality.

2. Essentially, the handbook proposes two routes for making time for patients. The first is to examine in detail the way wards work and, where necessary, *change* the way nurses spend time with and away from patients. On the majority of wards the Audit Commission looked at, the methods of organising nurses' work tend to fragment patient care. As a result, although individual patients have contact with many nurses, and individual nurses have contact with many patients, neither finds the contact satisfactory. Cumulatively, there is a great amount of patient-nurse contact, but because it is fragmented, both patients and nurses experience the latter as having very little time.

3. The second route is to review the management of the resources available for delivering care to patients, and again, to make changes if they are needed. Responsibility for the quality of patient care needs to be linked to control over ward resources, and vested as close to the ward as possible. This makes it easier to deploy *all* the resources of the ward effectively – including nursing and non-nursing staff time, the mix of skills and equipment – to meet the objectives for patient care.

4. In 1991, the Audit Commission published *The Virtue of Patients: Making Best Use of Ward Nursing Resources* (Ref.1) which gave an overview of the problems in delivering patient care, staffing wards and managing nursing services in hospital. It called for leadership at senior management level, support for 'bottom up' approaches to change-management and quality-improvement, and proposed a framework of action for senior managers to improve the service to patients.

HANDBOOK STRUCTURE

The handbook begins with a vision of the good quality nursing care it intends to promote, seen through the eyes of a patient and of a visitor to the ward, and sets out to show how it can be achieved.

— **Section 3** of the handbook gives the Audit Commission's criteria for assessing quality in nursing, and the reasons for them.

— **Section 4** uses the criteria to analyse the problems and difficulties that typically result in fragmented and non-patient-centred care.

— **Sections 5** gives practical examples from wards and hospitals to show how the problems and difficulties can be overcome.

— **Section 6** is about developing systems that allow for continuous improvements in the quality of patient care and managing the process of change.

5. The intention behind this second Audit Commission publication on acute nursing is to strengthen the 'bottom up' side of the equation by examining the process of delivering nursing care to patients, and describing in more detail the quality problems associated with it and the good practice solutions discovered in NHS hospitals.

6. It is written for that audience of key change agents close to the wards that is made up of nurses, ward sisters and charge nurses, nurses in what are variously described as 'quality' and 'resource management' posts, and middle managers positioned immediately above the wards. There is not a generic term that can sensibly be applied to the last group. There is too much variety in organisational structures and in the titles attached to posts at this level. But the managers close to the wards, often now carrying responsibility for a handful of wards or more within a Clinical Directorate or Unit, are ideally placed to put into effect the recommendations the Audit Commission made in *The Virtue of Patients* and to support the changes on the wards that are needed.

7. The research for the handbook was conducted in a representative sample of 10 NHS hospitals. The project team looked in detail at a sample of 39 general medical, general surgical and acute care of the elderly wards, visited wards in other hospitals to follow-up cases of good practice about which it had heard, and paid brief visits to hospitals in the USA and in France. The team was advised periodically during the course of its research by a panel of senior nurses, managers and academics and by a group of ward sisters and clinical nurse managers.

What is Good Quality Nursing Care?

INTRODUCTION

8. It would be difficult to overstate the psychological and emotional impact on patients of admission to hospital, even for those who by virtue of the frequency of their hospital stays eventually become 'expert patients'. On acute general wards, the majority of patients anticipate going into hospital more with relief than anxiety, but for a significant number the hospital stay is associated with major worries and fears (Exhibit 1). Those who are admitted in an emergency have no time to plan or to prepare themselves for their hospital stay. On general medical wards this applies to three quarters of the patients, and on general surgical wards, to more than one in three.

9. On every acute ward there are some patients for whom the stay in hospital comes to represent a turning point in their lives – either because their diagnosis or treatment affects their sense of their own identity, or because they have to change future plans. In this often unexpected, and always unwelcome position, they find themselves feeling psychologically as well as physically dependent on hospital staff, and especially vulnerable to the attitudes the professional staff take towards them.

10. The major surveys of patient opinion of the past twenty five years show that when they are in hospital, patients want to be on good terms with the professional staff; to be kept informed about their condition, treatment and progress; and to have a sense of being cared for personally rather than as a medical condition or 'a body in a bed'.

Exhibit 1

LEVELS OF PATIENT ANXIETY ON ACUTE GENERAL WARDS
One in five patients on acute general wards expresses major anxiety

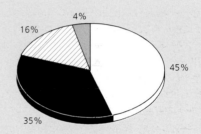

☐ 'I wasn't particularly bothered/ I wasn't at all worried'

■ 'I was nervous but not too anxious about going in'

▨ 'I was very worried about what might happen'

▦ 'I was expecting the worst'

Source: *Health Policy Advisory Unit*

THE PATIENT'S STORY

11. The text that follows is from an interview with a patient who had a very good experience on an acute surgical ward. She is a woman who has had a number of operations over a period of ten years, and in common with a great many of the patients one finds on all acute general wards, she has become an 'expert', able to compare the experience of a number of wards in different hospitals. In the interview she also talks about the patient in the next bed, an older woman admitted for major emergency bowel surgery.

Arriving on the ward

'When I arrived at the ward they told me I'd have to wait a while for a bed. I suppose I wasn't surprised, even though I had an appointment, but I thought 'oh no, this isn't a very good start...'. Whilst I was waiting in the corridor, the ward clerk came and introduced herself and told me what was happening. She said I'd be admitted as soon as they had a bed, and that one of the nurses – she called her 'your nurse' – would come and see me. I wasn't sure what she meant, but I felt better. At least they hadn't forgotten me.

Introductions and information

Once the bed was free, the clerk came and got me. She showed me to the bed... 'My nurse' was called Angela. She introduced herself, and made it clear she had enough time to talk. She just sat down on the bed next to me and waited. There were loads of questions I had forgotten to ask the doctor in out-patients, but I remembered most of them and she gave me answers. She explained what was going to happen and talked a lot about the anaesthetic and how I was likely to feel afterwards. It meant I could ask her about after the operation. I wasn't sure if I'd be able to drive, and she said it would be fine.

She also told me about the other nurses and who was going to look after me. She said she wouldn't be there after the operation and I wouldn't see her again before I went home because the next day was her day off. She asked me quite a bit about how I was going to get home. I had already made sure my husband would be around because of course I knew when I was coming out. She said the other nurse who would look after me was Jane and I should ask her if I was bothered about anything.

Names and identities

It was different from the other times I've been in hospital, in so many ways. I don't think a nurse has ever told me her name and sat down with me like that. I remember last time I was in hospital I actually called one of the nurses by her name. I'd seen it on her badge and I didn't want to just shout 'Nurse!' She looked so surprised and I still don't know if she thought I was a bit impertinent. You never do know, do you? To begin with I wasn't sure who the sister was this time. There was a nurse who seemed more senior and I saw her giving advice to another nurse. But when I got out of bed, I could see all the photographs on the wall, and she was the sister.

Flexible responses

When I came to after the operation I had missed supper completely and I was so hungry. This nurse, Jane, was there then, and when she saw I was awake she came and asked me how I was. She made me some tea and toast. The other thing that really impressed me and was so different… last time I was in hospital, do you know the night nurse actually woke me up to ask if I wanted a sleeping pill? It makes me laugh now. Well, I heard the night nurse this time – she was going round asking who wanted sleeping pills and pain killers – she said to one of the patients 'you need to tell me now, because I won't wake you later.' I woke up at 4.30 in the morning. Last time, I remember, you felt guilty if you woke up early, well before they woke you up, and I was actually told off for putting the light on. But when the night nurse saw I was awake, she came and asked how I was and offered me a cup of tea. She asked if I wanted the light on or to go the day room. But I had the tea and went back to sleep. When I woke up it was half past seven. Most people were awake, but they didn't wake everyone up. I suppose some people might have missed breakfast, but…sometimes you'd rather sleep if you feel awful. Don't you think so?

Allocation

My neighbour had been on the ward for nine days. She had been incredibly ill and had an operation that took seven hours the day she came in. She was walking around but she still felt dreadful. She had a different nurse, not Angela. She told *me the way it worked. She basically had three nurses who always looked after her and there were two students who worked with them. She said the students had all left the previous week, and all the students on the ward now were new. She liked it. She said she felt she could help the students in a way, and she didn't mind them looking after her because she knew there was a fully trained nurse supervising them.*

Discharge home

She had been very worried about going home. She lives with her youngest daughter who is twelve, her husband and her mother. They all came in to see her except the mother who isn't very well herself. What she was worried about was not being able to manage everything as soon as she went home. She almost didn't want to go home because she was so worried about how she'd cope. But her nurse had spoken to her about it and since then she had got over it. Her nurse had asked her husband to come in for an appointment with her and she had explained to him that his wife wouldn't be able to do everything and he'd have to help a bit more than usual. She felt he'd taken it from the nurse and really wanted to help.'

WHAT THE VISITOR SEES

12. Wards send signs and signals to the outside world about their values and priorities. Visitors to hospitals rapidly learn a great deal about wards from these signs: about the way they work, about the value the staff place on helping individual patients to feel at ease (if not at home) and, above all, on whether the service is there for the patient or the other way round. Some of the more important signs are:

Respect for the patient's privacy and dignity

There are enough screens in sufficiently good repair to protect adequately the privacy and dignity of every patient. Nurses are careful to use them at all times. Patients have the right size hospital night-gowns and pyjamas, and all the openings have fasteners that work. Visitors do not inadvertently overhear confidential matters being discussed between professional staff or with patients. Instead, they observe nurses taking time to answer patients' questions fully. When nurses do not know the answer to a question they can be heard promising to find out and report back later.

Written and visual information

The ward provides a variety of written and printed information to patients and their visitors. It is attractively produced, kept up to date and carefully displayed (see Figure 1 a,b). If there are notices for patients and staff, for example, it is evident from their position and sign-posting which are for the patients. Information is placed where patients can reach it. On one ward, for example, a leaflet about the ward is placed on every bedside locker. The information may include:

▼ Information handed to patients as they leave the ward. Patients are given written information about the drugs they take home, their next appointment at the hospital, health advice and a telephone number to contact if they should need it.

▼ The name of the doctor and the nurse who has overall charge of the patient's care posted at the head or foot of the bed where it is clear to see.

▼ Notices inviting patients to make suggestions and give feedback,

Figure 1(a)

WELCOME TO YORK GALLERY

We hope that your stay with us will be as comfortable as possible. We practise TEAM NURSING on this ward, this means that as far as possible you will be looked after by the same team of nurses throughout your stay with us. We want you to be involved in any decisions concerning your nursing care so please feel free to ask any questions, your nurses will be happy to answer them.

Sometimes (for various reasons) we have to move patients to another team. If this is the case you will be introduced to your new team and they will be made fully aware of your needs.

If you have any worries or complaints regarding your nursing care, please do not hesitate to discuss them with your nurses or the ward sisters.

Below is a list of all involved in your care:

your team of Nurses: ....
....
....
....
....
....

your Consultant: ....
your Senior Registrar: ....
your Registrar: ....
your Senior House Officer: ....

Our nursing philosophy is overleaf.

Source: Royal Brompton and National Heart Hospital, London

Figure 1 (b)

YOU CAN EXPECT YOUR PRIMARY NURSE TO:

Get to know you and your family.
Plan with your doctor, for your care.
Plan with you the nursing care, to meet your needs.
Explain your needs to the associate nurse, who will care for you
when your primary nurse is off duty.
Tell you what to expect before all tests or treatment.
Teach you about health care related to your condition.
Find the answers, to your questions, about your hospital stay.

WE NEED YOU TO:

Tell your primary nurse what you need.
Keep your nurse informed about how you feel and things that
are on your mind.
Let your nurse know how you feel about the care you receive.
Tell your nurse if you have an idea or a preference about your
nursing care.

Source: Tameside General Hospital, Ashton-under-Lyne

and giving them information about where and how to make complaints.

▼ Health education leaflets selected to meet the particular needs and interests of the patients normally on the ward.

▼ Up-to-date photographs, showing members of staff individually with their name and position clearly labelled. (Some wards display photographs of staff parties, but whilst the staff may enjoy looking at them they are very rarely helpful to patients.)

Communication

Nurses can be seen introducing themselves, and explaining what their role is to be in relation to the patient. They use plain English, avoid jargon and technical terms, stand around the head of the bed and speak loudly enough for the patient to hear what they have to say. They are careful not to discuss confidential or embarrassing matters in the hearing of other patients, but to leave these for discussion with the patient at a point when it is possible to have some privacy.

Explicit account of the religious and cultural requirements of patients represented in the local catchment population

The written information is available in languages other than English spoken in the local community, and arrangements for interpreters and patient advocates on the wards are clearly posted. Attention is clearly paid to the different dietary needs of patients, to the need for special arrangements for washing and clothing, and to any special requirements at time of death.

Ward philosophies

Tell patients and visitors what the ward is aiming to achieve and what they – the patients – can and should expect (see Figure 2 a,b). They are written in plain English, using expressions such as 'looking after every patient as an individual' instead of nursing terms like 'individualised patient care'. They are positioned where everyone can read them, usually at the entrance to the ward or near the door. Often they are written in large print and framed, which makes them attractive as well as easy to read.

Care plans

Nurses are to be seen writing care plans at the patient's bed rather than in the office, or at a table in the centre of the ward. This makes it easier for the patient to contribute to the plan and to ask questions about the record.

Handover

The handovers at the bedside genuinely include the patient. The maximum number of nurses is unlikely to be more than four.

Figure 2 (a)

WARD PHILOSOPHY

OUR AIM IS TO ENSURE THAT EACH PATIENT RECEIVES CARE OF THE HIGHEST STANDARD

Our patients will be regarded as individuals who have the right to make decisions regarding their own nursing care.

•••••••••••••••••

Nursing care will be aimed towards supporting the patient to meet his own personal needs or using a relative, friend or a nurse when this is not possible. All nursing care will be planned and carried out in partnership with the patient.

•••••••••••••••••

Each patient's care will be carried out by an individual nurse who will accept full responsibility for planning and carrying out the nursing care. He/she will be held accountable for the quality of nursing care given to the patient. Nursing actions will be continously evaluated and be based on the latest nursing research.

•••••••••••••••••

The nurse's role as a health educator will be recognised and encouraged. Patients will be given every opportunity to become well informed about their illness.

•••••••••••••••••

Nurses on York gallery will be encouraged to be responsible for their own professional development. They will be given the opportunity to apply for and attend educational, training course and seminars.

Figure 2 (b)

```
        PATIENT INFORMATION
     WELCOME TO VICTORIA WARD

TO IMPROVE PATIENT CARE AND ENSURE
CONTINUITY OF CARE BY THE NURSES
LOOKING AFTER YOU, TEAM NURSING IS
PRACTISED ON THIS WARD. THERE ARE 3
TEAMS ON THE WARD, EACH OF WHICH IS
LED BY A SENIOR STAFF NURSE. EACH
TEAM LOOKS AFTER A GROUP OF PATIENTS
AND ON ADMISSION TO THE WARD YOU
WILL BE ALLOCATED TO ONE OF THESE
TEAMS. THE NURSES WILL INTRODUCE
THEMSELVES AND WILL DISCUSS WITH YOU
HOW THEY CAN ASSESS, PLAN, IMPLEMENT
AND EVALUATE YOUR CARE THROUGHOUT
YOUR STAY. ALL OF THIS INFORMATION
WILL BE KEPT IN A YELLOW FOLDER AT
THE END OF YOUR BED WHICH YOU ARE
WELCOME TO READ,    AND CONTRIBUTE TO
YOUR  CARE.  YOUR    RELATIVES  AND
FRIENDS     ARE     ENCOURAGED    TO
PARTICIPATE IN YOUR CARE AS WELL.
FOR FURTHER INFORMATION PLEASE ASK
YOUR TEAM NURSES.


WE HOPE YOU WILL ENJOY YOUR STAY
WITH US.
```

Source: Royal Brompton and National Heart Hospital, London

13. Last, but not least, and of great significance given the title of this handbook, one of the signs that tells the visitor a great deal about the ward is its atmosphere. Where the individual patient is at the centre of nursing activity the atmosphere invariably appears to be calmer and less frenetic than on other wards. Nurses seem not to be rushing around looking so busy that it would have to be a brave patient indeed who asked for their attention. Nor do they sit in groups together, on the ward or in the office, recovering from the rush over cups of coffee and tea. Instead, the pace of their work appears to proceed more steadily. No doubt they are busy, but they appear more in control and the pace of work is more even. It is also more common to see them sitting with patients without necessarily 'doing' anything to or for them, simply sitting and talking.

3

General Problems with Definitions of Quality in Nursing

14. In health care generally, outcome measures are considered superior to other types of quality measure. But in nursing, as in every other area of clinical work, the relationship between patient outcomes and the activities of the nurses and other clinicians that may have produced them need to be clearly and precisely understood.

15. There is a great need for more research into clinical nursing practice, but the methodological problems in this area are severe.

▼ It is difficult to identify the part played by clinical treatment generally from what might be termed 'patient factors', such as the psychological and emotional support of friends and family.

▼ It is difficult to distinguish the specific contribution of *nursing* (as opposed to any other clinical discipline) to an individual patient's progress.

▼ Randomised control trials and case control experiments are not easy to mount in the extraordinary complexity of the environment of an acute general ward.

▼ The same standardisation problems occur in dealing with differences between individual patients as in all other areas of clinical research.

16. In nursing, it is arguably especially important to develop *measures of process* – that is, objective ways of describing and measuring what nurses do to patients and how they do it, because so much of what patients value about nursing is contained in the process. What patients care about is *how* nurses 'do nursing': *how* they respond when the patient calls out or makes a request; *how* they offer help with washing, sitting up in bed, moving from the bed, eating; *how* they answer questions, and so on.

Exhibit 2

PATIENTS' ASSESSMENTS OF THE DEGREE TO WHICH THEY ARE TREATED AS INDIVIDUALS IN HOSPITAL

One in four patients feels a lack of individual care and attention

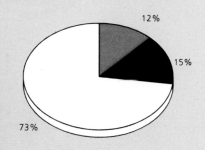

'I felt that whilst in hospital I was merely another body on a health conveyor-belt'

'At times I felt that I didn't receive the personal care and attention that I would have liked whilst in hospital'

'The attention I received was so personal in nature that I never felt that I had lost my individuality'

Source: Health Policy Advisory Unit

PUBLIC OPINION OF THE QUALITY OF NURSING CARE

17. Historically, the public has always rated nursing and nurses highly, but a number of recent surveys of patient opinion have demonstrated rising levels of dissatisfaction with hospital care in general, including nursing. The dissatisfaction centres upon the lack of personal care and the poor quality of patient-nurse communication. In relation to both, patients talk about nurses 'not having enough time for them.'

Personal care: Although most patients say they are well cared for in hospital, one in four says the care is impersonal and feels like a production line (Exhibit 2). In one survey, a third of the respondents who had been in hospital in the previous twelve months complained about the rigid timetable of the ward, being woken early and the poor quality of the meals. One in five said the nurses had been 'too busy to attend to their individual needs' (Ref. 2).

Patient-nurse communication: Between a quarter and a third of patients express dissatisfaction with their contact with professional staff. Although it is a minority who complain about nurses, one in five says nurses could try harder to make sure patients understand the information and that they leave the responsibility for information-giving to doctors (Exhibit 3). One sixth of the complaints about nursing care investigated by the Ombudsman in 1990-1991 were concerned with problems with communication (Ref. 3).

NURSING OPINION OF THE QUALITY OF NURSING CARE

18. It is not only the patients who regret the lack of individualised care and feel that 'nurses do not have enough time' for real communication. A number of recent surveys of nursing opinion have shown 'problems in delivering patient-centred care' are a significant factor contributing to low morale amongst nurses and a reason many nurses give for leaving NHS employment (Refs. 4, 5 and 6). Many nurses are dissatisfied with what they experience as a gap between the rhetoric of the nursing process which talks about 'individualised' or 'patient-centred care', and the reality of discontinuous and routinised patient care on acute general wards. Along with the patients, they too attribute the difficulties they have delivering patient care to 'not having enough time for the patients'.

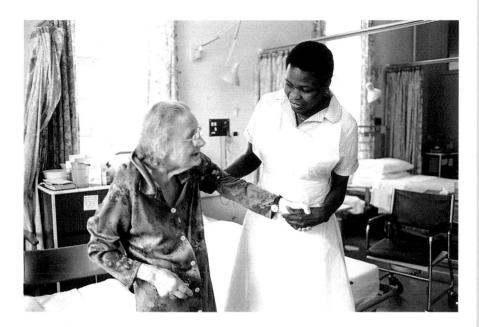

THE AUDIT COMMISSION'S CRITERIA FOR ASSESSING QUALITY OF NURSING CARE

19. The Audit Commission bases its assessment of quality in nursing on the degree to which the care succeeds in being (a) continuous and (b) centred on the needs of the individual patients (Box A, overleaf).

20. Continuity and patient-centred care are so fundamentally intertwined that it is difficult to say where one begins and the other ends. In order to see the benefits of detailed, individualised care planning, individual nurses need to have continuous relationships with individual patients. They need to witness the consequences for patients of nursing decisions. If their contact with individual patients is fragmented, they will find it more difficult to value care-planning and to devote to it the time it requires. Care plans are the key to providing continuity and personalised care. They are the vehicle that allows the many different nurses caring for the same patient to direct their work with that patient towards an explicit and agreed common goal.

Exhibit 3

PATIENTS' VIEWS OF COMMUNICATION WITH NURSES
One in five patients feel nurses could try harder to make sure they understand the information they are given

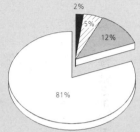

'The nurses:

- always left it to the doctors or medical support staff to explain things to me'

- should have taken greater pains to explain matters to me'

- made little attempt to make sure that I understood everything they told me'

- always ensured that whatever they told me was thoroughly explained' and 'were usually very good at explaining things to me'

Source:: Health Policy Advisory Unit

REASONS FOR CHOOSING CONTINUITY AND PATIENT-CENTRED CARE

Patient Preference: they satisfy the conditions for achieving good communication and personalised care.

Clinical Effectiveness: despite the paucity of research, there are clear signals from intensive care and care of patients with heart disease (Refs. 7 and 8); and management of post-operative pain (Ref. 9) that continuous, patient-centred care is clinically more effective.

Professional Values: in education, policy and practice, the nursing profession is committed to the concept of individualised 'patient-centred' care, based on the implementation of the nursing process (Refs. 10, 11, 12 and 13). The Department of Health Nursing Division's *Strategy for Nursing* identifies primary nursing as a form of organisation that can provide continuity and personalised care. *The Patient's Charter,* has similar objectives, and commits hospitals to developing systems of 'named nursing'.

4

Problems in the Delivery of Nursing Care

Note

At the end of each sub-section there is a 'Good Practice' reference in the margin indicating the relevant paragraphs and page numbers in section 5.

21. Part I of this section of the handbook examines four factors that detract from continuity of care:

    (a)   Methods of allocating patients to nurses

    (b)   Problems in clinical decision-making

    (c)   Communication problems

    (d)   Poor discharge planning

and two factors that inhibit patient-centred care:

    (e)   Poor documentation

    (f)   Rigid ward timetables

Part II looks behind the scenes at the reasons for them.

INTRODUCTION

22. On the majority of wards in the Audit Commission's sample, the methods used to organise care prevent nurses from giving continuous, personalised care to patients. Nurses and managers at all levels of the service often attribute poor quality to 'lack of nursing time' or 'lack of resources'. But the Audit Commission found no evidence of a systematic relationship between the quantity of resources available on wards and quality of patient care. On the whole, what distinguishes the wards that are succeeding in achieving greater continuity and more patient-centred care from others, is that they manage to use *all* their resources, including clerical and support staff time and equipment, to release nursing time for patients.

Exhibit 4

METHODS OF ALLOCATING PATIENTS TO NURSES

On the majority of wards, methods of allocation prevent stable relationships developing between individual nurses and patients

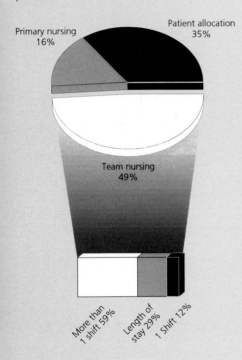

Primary nursing
16%

Patient allocation
35%

Team nursing
49%

More than
1 shift 59%

Length of
stay 29%

1 Shift 12%

Source: Audit Commission sample

---

23. In the majority of hospitals, it should be possible to improve the quality of care and create more nursing time for patients by changing the arrangements for managing the service to allow individuals at every level in the hierarchy to make the most of the opportunities. Management structures need to bring responsibility for the delivery of nursing care and control over the resources of the ward together and closer to the ward. The ward sister or manager (be it a nurse or a general manager) will then be well placed to make sure resources are used to their maximum to achieve care objectives.

24. Off the ward factors can detract from the quality of patient care. In particular, internal transfers of patients from one ward to another occurring for non-clinical reasons and caused by problems in bed management put continuity of care at risk. It is not usual for managers of nursing services to be in a position to prevent such moves. Ward-based nurses can try to 'contain the damage'– ensuring that the patients selected for transfer are suitable, that there is a proper handover to the receiving ward and that the patient's care plan goes too. But because the transfers themselves are not amenable to ward level solutions, this handbook does not discuss them. Readers are referred to the Audit Commission's report on acute bed management (Ref. 14) which makes a number of recommendations that can help to resolve problems at hospital level.

PART I

FACTORS DETRACTING FROM CONTINUITY OF CARE
(a) METHODS OF ALLOCATING PATIENTS TO NURSES

25. Methods of allocating patients to nurses determine the potential for stable individual patient-nurse relationships. On most sample wards, the Audit Commission found patients had very little sense of personal contact with individual nurses. The minority who confidently named *a nurse* responsible for their care (or one nurse 'and the others who work with her') were on wards that had explicitly identified continuity in individual patient-nurse relationships as a priority. These wards allocated the patient to the same nurses for the entire length of their stay.

26. The methods of allocation practised on the majority of wards prevent the development of stable patient-nurse relationships (Exhibit 4). Patients often do not know which nurse is looking after them. The feeling that all the nurses are in

some sense responsible creates uncertainty in their minds about which nurse to approach about serious worries or concerns.

27. One patient described how she felt about not knowing whether any of the nurses was 'hers'. She was particularly conscious of the difficulty because she had been in intensive care for seven days where she had been allocated to the care of one nurse in particular. Asked what she did when she needed help or wanted to talk to a nurse, she said:

> 'It's a case of who's passing at the time. It's very different here from in intensive care. Maybe I was spoilt, but here it's like walking into another world. You ask anybody, whereas there you know who's looking after you...I'm not all that impressed. I don't want to be uncharitable, but there seems to be a lack of interest in the individual. I mean we are all ill and you want a bit of pampering, but you don't get it.'

28. Many wards that describe themselves as doing 'team nursing' will be able to increase continuity of patient care and develop more stable relationships between patients and nurses by:

▼ Defining the nursing team's workload in terms of patients rather than beds.

This will allow patients who have to be moved to a different bed in the same ward to remain with the team that admits them.

▼ Not allowing teams to change ends at pre-determined intervals.

Teams change ends at intervals that last anything from three months to three days – a system that gives precedence to the needs of staff rather than patients. Indeed, on many wards where changing ends is routine, sisters feel obliged to provide nurses with 'variety' and to share out the less popular patients amongst the staff.

But changing ends can prevent nurses from getting to know patients well enough to understand and empathise with their problems. And without that level of understanding, they will continue to see not 'patients with problems' (that are potentially amenable to solutions), but 'problem patients'.

▼ Compiling separate duty rosters for each team rather than one roster for the whole ward.

The single duty roster makes it more difficult to create stable team membership.

29. It is difficult to see any potential for stable relationships between individual nurses and patients on the wards currently doing patient allocation. As a method of organising care it permits individual patients to be looked after by different configurations of nurses on every shift. And it offers no guarantee to nurses that having worked with a patient on one shift, they will work with the same patient again.

(b) CLINICAL DECISION-MAKING

30. It is very difficult to generalise about clinical decision-making in nursing. All kinds of clinical decisions are made whilst patients are in hospital. Making such decisions is a highly complex activity that will be determined in part by major factors such as the stability of the patient's condition and dependency level. But it is useful to distinguish between the major decisions that will be made in the original care plan and whenever there is a need to reassess the main elements of the plan

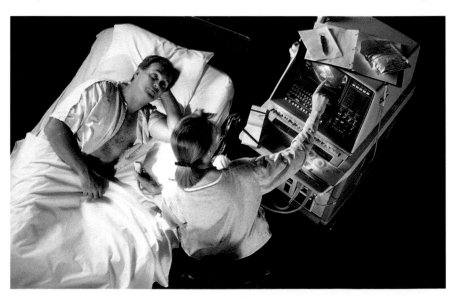

in a fundamental way, and the more immediate, minor decisions nurses make whilst they are in contact with patients. Which nurses are involved in making the different types of decision will depend on the system for organising care and the ward sister's judgement of the experience and competence of members of the ward nursing team. She will decide who is ready to take responsibility for individual patients' care.

31. Because nursing is a 24-hour a day activity and individual nurses work shifts lasting anything from 7.5 to 12 hours, the degree to which there is continuity in the decision-making process will depend upon:

▼ The number of nurses making decisions about individual patients.

The greatest continuity is achieved on wards where the responsibility for planning the care of individual patients, and for major reassessments of the plan, is delegated to one trained nurse – either the primary nurse or the leader of a team – for the length of the patient's stay.

A third of the Audit Commission sample wards attempt to limit the number of nurses who might potentially be involved in decisions about an individual patient to those in the patient's team. But half set no limits to the numbers of nurses who can make decisions about the care of an individual patient (Exhibit 5). Any nurse on duty and available at the time of the patient's admission will complete the initial assessment and plan of care and any other nurse working with that patient on a subsequent shift evaluates and updates the plan (including the discharge plan).

▼ The amount of direct contact between the nurse(s) who make the decisions and the patient.

There is more continuity when the nurse who makes the decisions is directly involved in caring for the patient.

Traditionally, the ward sister provided continuity by making all the major decisions. But many sisters now feel they spend very little time with patients and they are increasingly less involved in clinical care. Logically, this means that if they are continuing to take responsibility

Exhibit 5

RESPONSIBILITY FOR PATIENT ASSESSMENT AND MAJOR DECISIONS IN NURSING CARE
On half the wards there is very little continuity in clinical decision-making

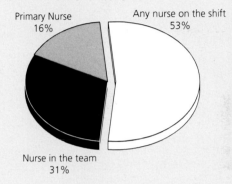

Primary Nurse 16%
Any nurse on the shift 53%
Nurse in the team 31%

Source: Audit Commission sample

for clinical decision-making the decisions are being made by someone with comparatively little first-hand knowledge of the patients.

▼ The degree of clarity about who is responsible for individual patients.

The wards where everyone – staff and patients – knows who is responsible for particular patients, are the minority mentioned above where responsibility for making major decisions about individual patients is clearly delegated to either a primary nurse or a team leader. But on other wards, there is a considerable amount of confusion about the roles of ward sisters and trained nurses and the responsibility for individual patients.

On patient allocation wards and most team nursing wards, sisters feel responsible for what they describe as the 'most important' decisions, leaving the less important to the nurses delivering care to the patient. But because there is very little discussion about the criteria for judging the relative importance of different types of decision, and a considerable amount of anxiety about delegation, nurses and patients are effectively in a kind of 'no-man's-land' in which everyone, or no-one, might be making decisions.

32. In most hospitals, nurses have been left to develop their own interpretation of the terms 'accountability' and 'responsibility', and have arrived at their own definitions. Many sisters are not certain that it is possible to retain overall responsibility for the care of patients on their wards whilst delegating the responsibility for individual patients to other nurses. They are also uncertain about how to square the idea of delegation with the UKCC's requirement that its members should be accountable at all times for their practice.

33. Nurses and managers at every level need to clarify together the distinction between overall responsibility for patient care delivered on wards (including responsibilities for cover, for standards and for making sure every patient has an individual plan of care); responsibility for the decisions that need to be made in the care of individual patients; and accountability for one's own practice. Once these distinctions have been thoroughly understood, it should be possible for sisters to delegate responsibility for clinical decisions to other qualified members of staff.

Good Practice

— (b) Clinical Decision-making.
Paragraphs 77-78, pages 36-37

(c) COMMUNICATION

34. Building continuity in patient-nurse relationships, and clarifying who is responsible for the care of individual patients will improve the communication between nurses and patients, and between nurses and their colleagues from other professions.

Communication between patients and nurses

35. On primary nursing and some team nursing wards, patients and their visitors are encouraged to share information and direct questions to the primary nurse or team leader. Elsewhere, they are left to make up their own minds about the 'right' channels of communication. They have to try and decide for themselves whether to talk to the nurse they see most frequently, the nurse looking after them at the moment, the ward sister, or the nurse they like best.

36. Sometimes nurses complain that patients give information to the 'wrong' person, meaning domestic staff and very junior students. They need to understand how difficult it is for patients to know (without being told) who is the 'right' person.

Communication between nurses at handover

37. Although nurses communicate with each other all the time, the shift handover is a critical moment as far as maintaining continuity is concerned.

38. Wards vary considerably in how they conduct handovers and there do not appear to be any strict rules. The Audit Commission sample divides almost equally between office and bedside handovers. Theoretically, bedside handovers allow greater patient participation, but how much the patient is really able to participate will depend less on where the handover takes place than on the approach and the skills of the nurses. Some bedside handovers are reminiscent of medical ward rounds and involve patients comparatively little.

39. Measures that diminish the risk of losing continuity of individual patient's care at handover are:

▼ Making sure the nurse making the report has direct, first-hand knowledge of the patient, and is not relying on other nurses' reports for information.

Good Practice

— Communication between patients and nurses. Paragraphs 79-80, page 38

▼ Keeping written information about the patient in one place and avoiding duplication.

On many wards, information about the same patient is held in a number of different places – the care plan; checklists; the Kardex; the ward diary; the notes the nurses make for themselves and keep in their pocket.

▼ Valuing the written patient record.

Only a minority of wards make constructive use of the written records at handover and expect nurses on the in-coming shift to read them. Most place much more importance on oral communication, but this means that any nurse not present at the handover is deprived of access to the information.

▼ Not using up the handover time by repeating the standard information about patients that nurses can get from the notes (name, age, diagnosis), but taking the time to discuss individual patients and their care more fully, and in greater depth.

Communication between nurses and other health professionals

40. Inter-professional communication is a top priority for everyone in hospital. Nurses and their professional colleagues from other disciplines place great store by multi-disciplinary meetings and acute care of the elderly wards are particularly good at organising them. Two thirds of the wards hold regular meetings, although members of the other professions, and doctors in particular often do not attend.

41. Communication works best when there is agreement about the correct channels, mutual respect, and a common basis for discussion, i.e. first-hand knowledge of the patient. Gaps in communication and misunderstandings between health professionals are not only detrimental to patient care, they also affect the communication between professional and patient adversely.

42. Many wards are changing the way nurses communicate with professional colleagues from other disciplines. Traditionally, the ward sister has been *the* person who communicates with the doctors and all the other professional staff, but increasingly that responsibility is being devolved to the nurse who is responsible for the patient. On almost twenty-five per cent of sample wards, for example, the

Good Practice

— Communication between nurses at handover. Paragraph 81, pages 38-39 team leader or the primary nurse for the specific patient attends the consultant's ward round.

43. On some wards, nurses have made changes in the way they work without discussion with their immediate colleagues. Where the tensions and difficulties surrounding the changes are particularly acute, they sometimes need to spend more time discussing and explaining in advance what they are trying to do, to help their colleagues understand.

44. Other health professionals witness the changes in the role of the sister, and often seem to interpret them in terms of loss: loss of authority; loss of status; loss of contact; loss of interest and, some say, loss of commitment to nursing. Significantly, many of them identify with the sister's perceived losses and feel undermined themselves if a more junior nurse than the sister deals with them. One consultant, for example, feels the sister allows junior nurses to accompany him on his round because she does not value contact with doctors.

(d) DISCHARGE PLANNING

45. Good discharge planning is essential for continuity of care.

▼ There is a need for clarity about who has overall responsibility for the patient's discharge plan.

On many wards, the ward sister is nominally responsible, but the implementation of the plan is handed on from one nurse to the next with each change of shift. No one person is ever fully responsible for all aspects of the plan.

▼ Responsibility for communicating with the patient, the patient's close relatives and with professional colleagues needs to be clearly established.

Nurses on the wards, and visiting professional staff – such as the social worker, the community liaison nurse and the physiotherapist – need to know who to talk to about each individual patient's discharge plan, and how to reach them.

Good Practice

— Communication between nurses and other health professionals. Paragraphs 82-83, pages 40

Exhibit 6

NURSES' ANSWERS TO THE QUESTION
Most hospitals have a discharge policy but
staff on the wards do not know of it or regard
it as of little practical use

'Does your hospital have a discharge policy'

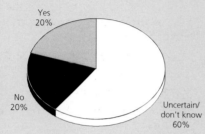

Yes
20%

No
20%

Uncertain/
don't know
60%

Source: *Audit Commission interviews on sample wards*

Exhibit 7

**NURSES' DESCRIPTIONS OF WHERE THE
DISCHARGE PLAN IS KEPT**
Information relating to the patient's discharge
is kept in more than one place

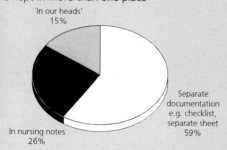

'In our heads'
15%

Separate
documentation
e.g. checklist,
separate sheet
59%

In nursing notes
26%

Source: *Audit Commission interviews on sample wards*

Good Practice

— (d) Discharge planning.
Paragraphs 84-86, pages 41-45

▼ Documentation: it is helpful to document assessments for discharge planning and discharge plans in full, and to include mention of the views and feelings of patients and their relatives.

It is also useful to simplify the documentation so that anyone wanting to check the plan, knows where to find it. Information relating to the patient's discharge is often kept in more than one place: in case-notes, ward diaries, the ward clerk's lists of duties for the day and, most problematically, in nurses' heads (Exhibit 6).

▼ Discharge policies and procedures.

Although nurses and managers seem more than convinced of the importance of discharge planning, only two out of ten hospitals in the Audit Commission sample had accompanied the introduction of a new discharge policy and procedures with awareness training. Six of the ten hospitals had policies staff had either not seen, or found to be of little practical use (Exhibit 7). Two hospitals had no discharge policy at all. None of the hospitals had systems in place for monitoring discharges or discharge planning.

46. The current solutions to the problems in this area tend to be superficial and cosmetic. They most frequently take the form of checklists, new stationery or newly designed documentation. They generally do not make much impact because they tend to tackle the symptom leaving the root cause of the problem – the organisation of care – untouched.

FACTORS INHIBITING PATIENT-CENTRED CARE
(e) PLANNING PATIENT CARE

47. Written needs assessment and care plans are the practical medium through which the care of patients is 'individualised'. Writing care plans and maintaining the records takes time. On one primary nursing ward where the care-planning and record-keeping was thorough and detailed, the trained nurses estimated that they spent up to twenty per cent of their time on this activity.

48. The Audit Commission's examination of patient records confirms the Ombudsman's view of record-keeping in nursing as 'ritualistic', and lacking essential information (Box B) (Ref. 3).

49. Nurses need greater incentives to invest the time and energy that care planning requires. Specifically, they need to be able to feel the benefits of doing it properly. They need to be able to develop professionally through writing comprehensive, detailed care plans, seeing the outcomes of their own clinical decisions, learning from their mistakes, and judging the quality of their planning skills. Often their involvement with individual patients is too brief and intermittent. They do not see the same patient more than once, and very few see the patient right through to the end of the hospital stay. On ten per cent of the sample wards, the care planning process is so fragmented that one nurse assesses the patient and a different nurse writes the plan of care.

50. Many ward sisters recognise the need to improve record-keeping and care planning, but have not themselves had the experience of seeing it done well. They need to develop confidence in their own abilities to develop the planning and written skills on the nursing team, and support from their medical colleagues who are sometimes openly dismissive of what they regard as nurses wasting time 'form-filling'.

51. Some wards are experimenting with different methods of improving care planning. These include multi-disciplinary care planning; sending nurses on courses; re-designing stationery; introducing core care plans or standardised care plans for common medical and nursing problems; and investing in computerised care planning systems. It is unusual to find wards where innovations of this kind are routinely evaluated. The tendency instead is to herald any change as necessarily an improvement, and to stick with it until the next one comes along. None of the solutions has proved wholly successful, nor are they likely to, until methods of organising the delivery of nursing care build continuity into the relationships between individual patients and nurses.

PROBLEMS WITH NURSING RECORDS
— records undated and unsigned
— lack of detail about the person rather than the medical problem
— insufficient information about the patient's perception of the problem, and response to treatment
— patient's psychological and emotional needs not documented
— objectives for care not established
— progress towards care objectives not evaluated
— assessments for discharge and discharge plans not documented

Good Practice

— (e) Planning patient care. Paragraph 87, page 46

(f) THE PATIENT'S DAY

52. The timetable of the patient's day can be a reliable indicator of the degree to which nursing care is led by the needs of individual patients as opposed to ward routines.

53. One of the most common complaints about hospitals is about being woken, and woken early. Ten per cent of sample wards allow patients to wake in their own time. A third of the wards wake them before 6.30 a.m.; the rest before 7.30 a.m. Once awake, patients sometimes wait up to two hours for breakfast.

54. But waking times apart, nurses on some wards still organise the patient's day around a set of routine activities that take place at times determined by the ward rather than the patient. This kind of system allows little or no room to take account of the different needs and preferences of individual patients.

55. The rationale for waking patients early and for delivering care on the basis of routines usually has to do with ideas about the amount of work needing to be done on different shifts. Often it is connected to managers' and nurses' desire to divide the work more evenly between the night and day shifts. Patients are woken, and sometimes turned and washed by night staff so that nurses on the early shift will not have to do it. Occasionally some patients do need to be woken early for clinical reasons, but this need not apply to the whole ward. Where ward sisters and their staff have wanted to move away from rigid timetables and early waking, they have found it possible to identify specific patients who need waking and make provision for them.

Good Practice

— (f) The patient's day. Paragraph 88, pages 46-47

Summary of Part I

The main problems in the delivery of patient care at ward level are linked to the essential activities of the nursing team:

— allocating patients to nurses;

— making clinical decisions;

— communicating with the patient and with professional colleagues;

— planning the patient's discharge from the ward;

— documenting the patient's care.

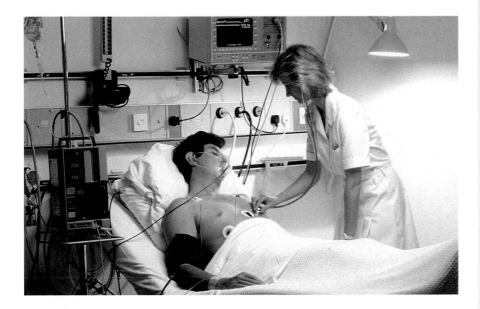

PART II

MANAGEMENT PROBLEMS UNDERLYING THE DELIVERY OF NURSING CARE

56. The factors that detract from continuity and patient-centred care cannot, as it were, simply be 'put right' by making one-off practical adjustments to the organisation of care. There is a need to return to the fundamentals of sound nursing, to ask 'who is the service for?', and to make sure that the answer is 'for the patient'. It is also important for nursing services to become more responsive and flexible so that they are continuously able to adapt to change: in the nature of the clinical work, in the individual and collective needs of patients, and in the organisation of health services.

57. There are three underlying problems in the management of nursing services that affect the quality of the care delivered to patients:

▼   a lack of systematic approaches to quality assessment and quality improvement;

▼   a need to bring responsibility for care and control of ward resources much closer together;

QUALITY ASSURANCE IN NURSING
Most wards do not have a systematic
approach to quality improvement and do not
routinely evaluate changes

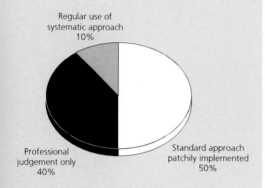

Regular use of
systematic approach
10%

Professional
judgement only
40%

Standard approach
patchily implemented
50%

Source: Audit Commission sample

▼   a need for greater clarity in management roles and relationships, particularly those of ward sisters and their immediate superiors.

58. Four brief case studies at the end of Part II illustrate the complex relationship that exists between the conduct of management and the delivery of patient care.

THE NEED TO PAY MORE SYSTEMATIC ATTENTION TO QUALITY

59. Systematic quality assessment is potentially one of the most valuable resources for developing practice and helping nursing staff to change. But whilst most hospitals routinely collect data on drug errors, accidents and falls, and some also collect data on hospital acquired infections and pressure sores, the data is put to limited use. Instead of being used in a systematic way to identify problems that might be occurring over time, with staffing, with ward management and with methods of organising patient care, it is more commonly used to find fault with individuals and apportion blame. Ward-based nurses rarely receive feedback about the data, and tend to see it as information 'for the hospital' or 'for them'. The same goes for educational audits which provide a wealth of comparative information about wards within the same hospital but which are rarely seen or used as quality assessment tools.

60. Instead, nurses rely heavily on their professional judgement to assess quality and on teaching to improve it. The most frequent types of quality related activity are: study sessions; audit meetings; quality circles; Total Quality Management meetings; and reviews using off-the-shelf audit packages such as MONITOR or QUALPACS (Exhibit 8). In five of the ten sample hospitals there is some quality related activity, but it tends to be fragmented and patchy. Standards are set but they are not monitored: a MONITOR exercise happens once, but is not repeated; or sisters attend study sessions on standard setting, and there is no follow-up.

61. Wards need to approach quality improvement systematically, and routinely to evaluate changes in nursing practice, in ward organisation and in the delivery of care. They need to obtain feedback from patients about their view of the service. And nurses need to begin to join together with colleagues from other health professions to develop clinical audit and multi-disciplinary standards of care.

62. Only a small minority of sisters and managers feel 'quality' is the 'flavour of the month' with general managers and a waste of time, or experience it as a direct attack on their professionalism. Most want feedback in the form of regular, objective information on the quality of care but lack confidence in their own abilities to set standards or introduce methods to improve quality. Invariably, they welcome help when it is made available.

THE SPLIT BETWEEN RESPONSIBILITY FOR THE WARD AND CONTROL OVER RESOURCES

63. Historically, responsibility for ward resources and for the clinical activity that takes place on the ward has tended to be split between the managers above the ward and outside it who have the resources (often a nurse manager controlling nursing, a medical records manager controlling administrative support, someone else managing the domestic staff, and so on) and the ward sister who is responsible for patient care. But many hospitals are now developing decentralised management structures that heal the divisions and bring the two much closer together.

64. The historical split made it difficult for anyone in the nursing hierarchy to make the links that need to be made to make sure all the resources are used in the best way possible to achieve good quality care. Managers outside the ward have had the final say in staff appointments and shift times, and the authority to move staff around the hospital. Many have 'kept an eye' on ward budgets without having the authority to move money between budget heads and change grade mix. Decisions about the size and composition of ward nursing establishments have often been made right at the top of the nursing hierarchy, without either the ward sister or the ward manager taking part.

65. Although formally, nurses at grade G and above have complete 24-hour a day responsibility for clinical care and the ward, their control over ward resources varies between hospitals, and in some cases, between wards in the same hospital.

▼ Most have some say over appointments to their own wards.

▼ Two out of three have authority over the start and end times of shifts and/ or the staff grade mix, but not the ordering of bank or agency staff, the size of the ward establishment or the budget.

Good Practice

— The need to pay more systematic attention to quality
Paragraphs 92-94, pages 48-51

▼ One in three has no authority or influence over shifts, grade mix, the size and composition of the establishment, or the budget.

▼ In fifty per cent (five out of ten) of sample hospitals a night nurse manager recruits and manages night staff and the ward sister does not control the nurses who work on her ward at night. The management of night nursing staff is under review in a great many hospitals with the responsibility gradually being transferred to the ward sister. But even where sisters manage their own night staff, those nurses can be re-deployed by night managers to other wards.

▼ Two out of three manage clerical staff, a smaller number manage domestic staff. But even where sisters have formal responsibility for support staff, they seem not to feel in control. In the ward clerk's absence, cover is almost never provided, and although one of the most common complaints is that nurses spend too much time on clerical and other 'non-nursing' duties, very few sisters negotiate changes in the amount of clerical time or in the actual hours the clerk works.

▼ Two of the sample hospitals call sisters 'budget holders'. In one, they simply monitor the budget, whilst in the other they have the power to move money between budget-heads and they participate in budget-setting meetings.

▼ Only a handful of sisters take part in meetings to set ward establishments.

THE LACK OF CLARITY IN MANAGEMENT ROLES AND RELATIONSHIPS

66. The profound changes in nursing and hospital management of the past decade have exposed nurse managers to a great deal of uncertainty about the expectations of others above and below them in the hierarchy. But although there is anxiety amongst managers and ward sisters about the concept of the 'ward manager', and about further and continuing changes in nursing management, some are thriving.

67. Many nurse managers are functioning with new titles or are in entirely new posts in structures that have not yet settled down. Whilst some lack a sense of achievement and feel guilty about 'spreading themselves too thinly', others have been able to turn this into an opportunity to develop new management skills or enter external courses of study for further qualifications (e.g. DMS and MBA).

They find the experience all the more worthwhile when there are other managers from the same hospital also on the course.

68. At ward sister level the same kind of differences obtain. Some ward sisters relish new and expanded roles and the opportunity to have more power to control the ward resources. But the pressures are intense and some can only describe their role as a list of responsibilities they struggle to meet: for patient care, teaching, and ward administration, staff development, and 'management' (meaning time away from the ward in management meetings).

69. Amongst the great variety of different accounts of the roles that sisters struggle to reconcile, there are four that prevail:

(i)   The *traditional* ward sister – who knows everything and everybody on the ward, makes all the decisions in clinical care and management of the ward, has immense personal authority and is respected by patients, nurses and medical staff alike. Paradoxically, perhaps, she has her shadow in the traditional image of the sister as someone who rules the ward from the office, has minimal direct contact with patients, is rarely seen out on the ward, and spends much of her time on routine administration.

(ii)   The ward sister as *clinical nurse*, struggling to retain a foot-hold in patient care, at odds with what she feels to be the illegitimate calls on her time that take her away from patients and students. One said *'I have less and less hands-on experience as a nurse. I've abandoned formal teaching because of the pressure. I'd like to spend more time with patients and students, and so I usually do the paperwork at home.'* Another described herself as 'a clinical person' who had never wanted to be away from patients. She resented the workload assessment system in use in the hospital, which she interpreted as evidence of senior managers' lack of faith in nurses' professional judgement: *'It's all dependencies and writing down'*.

(iii)   The sister as *manager-administrator*, who prioritises staff development, teaching and administration. Regardless of whether or not she is counted on the off-duty, she wants to spend less time on clinical care and devote more time to these activities. *'We're supposed to be managers and respon-*

sible for the ward', one said, '*so I spend all my time at work, and some out of it, with the staff. They need lots of support all the time, so I do my paperwork at home*'. Another, who described herself as '*teacher and leader of a team*', saw the principal needs governing her role as those of staff and students.

(iv) The sister as *manager-leader* who wants to be less involved in doing the work than in constructing the framework for it. This image of the sister is closely associated with the professional ideal of leading a team of practising professionals. Her role is to manage the wards, provide clinical expertise if required, set standards and monitor them, assess the skills and abilities of the the nurses and lend support where it is needed. One sister who had adopted this interpretation of the role said, '*If I'm not here, nothing should change. I see myself as the 'voice of the ward', negotiating between staff and management. I co-ordinate what goes on, but I don't usually do hands-on care myself*'.

Good Practice

— The lack of clarity in management roles and relationships. Paragraphs 95-104, pages 51-53

THE NEED TO MATCH RESPONSIBILITY FOR PATIENT CARE WITH CONTROL OF RESOURCES: FOUR CASE STUDIES

Case Study A

A ward sister organised the roster to support the development of primary nursing teams. But her attempt to create stability in her teams was undermined by hospital policy which dictated that temporary nurses should not work in the same area on more than three successive occasions. The hospital relied heavily on temporary staff and the policy was intended to reduce expenditure in this area. All requests for bank or agency nurses had to be channelled through one of the managers. Almost every time the sister needed temporary staff, a new bank nurse, unfamiliar with the ward and with the permanent members of the ward team, arrived on duty. In one month, this ward employed a different bank nurse on 80 separate shifts.

Case Study B

A ward sister wanting to introduce primary nursing needed another trained nurse on the team. Neither she nor her immediate manager were sure when or how the ward establishment was decided, who had the authority to change the grade mix or who controlled the ward budget. The sister's confidence in her own abilities to make changes and lead the nursing team was undermined and she became dispirited about both her position and her own management ability.

Case Study C

At the behest of management a ward conducted its own activity analysis which showed that nurses were spending over a quarter of their time on 'non-nursing' duties. The analysis showed that most of this time was spent answering the telephone, matching test results to medical notes and ordering supplies. As a result of the survey no action was taken. The clerical in-put to the wards was provided from the medical records budget (the medical records officer managed the ward clerks), and managers in nursing did not feel able to pursue the matter.

Case Study D

To build greater flexibility into the timetable of patients' days, a ward needed to vary the times at which nurses arrived on duty in the morning. The ward sister believed that she did not have the authority to change shift times and that hospital policy demanded standard shifts. Nevertheless, she placed a request with her manager to be allowed to stagger the start-times of some nurses. Her manager was unsure of her own authority in this area and passed the request up the tree to her manager. Although the sister had been waiting more than six months for an answer the manager felt unable to pursue the application on her behalf, sensing that her immediate superiors had 'more important' things on their minds. At the top of the nursing hierarchy, the Director of Nursing Services believed she had delegated managerial authority over shifts and grade mix to managers immediately above ward level.

Overcoming the Obstacles

INTRODUCTION

70. The two final sections of the handbook describe measures that will help nursing staff to deliver continuous, patient-centred care. Section 5 makes practical and technical recommendations that will make it possible for nursing staff to respond more easily to the individual needs of patients. Section 6 explores the structure and style of nursing management that can help to resolve the fundamental organisational problems underlying the delivery of nursing care on acute general wards. All the recommendations are based on methods of work and approaches to care that exist and are being tried in NHS hospitals.

71. Both sets of recommendations are important. The immediate problems in nursing on acute general wards are associated with a lack or loss of continuity and personalised care. But, inevitably, the problems of today will give way to new and different problems in the future. Advances in medical practice and technology, changes in the organisation of health services, and changes in the health status of populations, create a constant momentum with which nursing must keep pace.

72. The practical recommendations in this section are not intended as ready made solutions to the problems in any hospital or ward. Changing the delivery of nursing care is not an 'all or nothing' activity. It is an incremental process. Every ward is at its point somewhere along the quality dimensions; most achieve some but not all the criteria.

73. In every setting, it is important to take stock of the existing state of play, and to establish priorities specific to that setting. The plans will be implemented more effectively if nursing staff are able to make changes gradually at a manageable pace. More importantly, real and tangible improvements in the quality of patient care on acute general wards only come about when both the care objectives, and the

process of moving towards them, engages the imagination and aspirations of ward nurses.

74. It is possible that some recommendations will appear threatening, because they are about process – the 'how' of nursing – and about working practices. It is always important for the main change agents (in this case, managers and sisters) to prepare themselves in advance to encounter resistance – albeit passive resistance of the cynical variety. It is not unusual, for instance, to hear nurses insisting that there simply are not any wards practising 'real', stable, team / primary /named nursing, that claims to that effect are false, and that changing the organisation of care cannot be done without additional resources.

75. Leadership of the change process is essential, but it should not be seen as a mysterious quality that belongs to only a few chosen individuals. In hospital nursing, for example, it is associated with an accumulation of specific skills and experience put to good effect. The practical skills of the leading sisters and managers in the Audit Commission study lie in their own deep-seated knowledge of the clinical areas they manage, in planning, careful preparation, understanding what is going on and how patients and staff feel about it, sensitivity to timing and good judgement. The most effective leaders are experts in timing, knowing when to set new objectives, when to increase the pressure or quicken the pace, when to ease off to give time to consolidate and celebrate what has been achieved.

STRENGTHENING CONTINUITY OF CARE
(a) METHODS OF ALLOCATING PATIENTS TO NURSES

76. The number of nursing staff working with an individual patient on a ward needs to be kept to a minimum.

A variety of mechanisms help to reduce the numbers of nursing staff in contact with individual patients.

▼   The patient can be allocated to a named nurse who is a primary nurse and who has identified associates working with her patients on the shifts when she does not work. In this instance, only the primary nurse and her associates deliver direct care to the patient.

▼ Alternatively, the patient can be allocated to a team, with one member of the team nominated as the named nurse. Only nurses belonging to the team will be directly involved in caring for the patient.

▼ Once a patient has been allocated to a team, he/she remains with that team until their discharge from the ward.

▼ The roster is used as a tool to create stable sub-groups of nurses (primary nurse plus associates or teams). Within the sub-groups, nurses work on opposite shifts across the twenty-four hour period. Normally, this means abandoning the traditional form of hierarchical roster that is compiled for the ward as a whole, in favour of a roster that divides the total ward complement up into the requisite number of sub-groups. Each of the sub-groups is then conceptualised as a 'mini-ward', and rostered accordingly.

▼ The principle of reducing the numbers of different people in contact with individual patients is applied to student nurses, nursing auxiliaries and temporary staff. They are attached either to a primary nurse or to a team, and work with the patients belonging to that sub-group of nurses rather than with all the patients on the ward.

▼ On wards where the lay-out or restricted availability of piped gases makes it necessary to move patients around the ward, patients who have to be moved continue to be looked after by the same nurses. It can be a useful exercise to study the reasons for moving patients over a specified period of time. Frequently, it is habit of mind, the *idea* that acutely ill patients must be positioned directly in front of the nursing station, and not clinical necessity, that causes a move. Once nurses begin to develop stable relationships with patients it begins to seem more natural to take the care to the patient, than to move the patient to the care.

(b) CLINICAL DECISION-MAKING

77. Responsibility for clinical decisions in the care of individual patients is limited to nurses whose knowledge of the patient is acquired first-hand.

78. There is more than one way to increase continuity in clinical decision-making. However, the key to reducing the numbers of nurses involved in making clinical

decisions about individual patients and achieving clarity in the decision-making process is *delegation*.

▼ One nurse has *overall* responsibility for the assessment of the patient's needs, the plan of care, implementation and major evaluation of the plan throughout the patient's stay. This is the patient's named nurse, who may be a primary nurse or the leader of a team. The responsibility for decision-making does not pass from one nurse in charge to another with every shift, although clearly, the responsibility for providing safe care does.

▼ The deputising arrangements for decision-making when the responsible nurse is not on duty, including at night-time, are established clearly, and in advance.

▼ The patient and the patient's visitors, friends and relatives are told which nurse has this responsibility and they are encouraged to discuss any matters of concern with her. They are also told about the deputising arrangements.

▼ The name of the responsible nurse is written above the patient's bed and in other appropriate places.

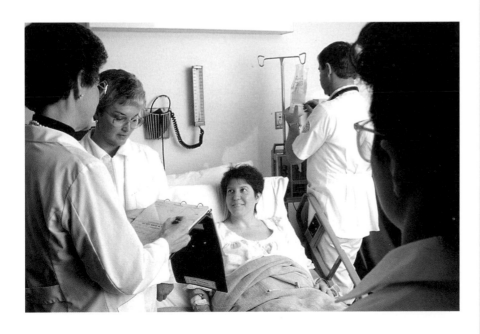

(c) COMMUNICATION

79. As a general rule, the number of people communicating with and about individual patients is kept to a minimum.

Communication between patients and nurses

80. The nurse who delivers care directly to the patient is responsible for communicating with the other health professionals involved in his or her care.

▼ Every patient is told the name of the nurse who has overall responsibility for the decisions in his or her care.

▼ The responsible nurse introduces herself by name, explains her role and makes sure the patient understands that if s/he is anxious or worried about anything, she is the person to tell.

▼ Every member of ward staff in contact with the patient for the first time introduces him or herself by name, explains who they are and their role in relation to the patient.

▼ Patients are given written information about the ward and the system of care, and invited to make suggestions and complaints.

Communication between nurses at handover

81. Because the method of allocation allows nurses to develop relationships with individual patients over time, the nurse arriving on duty (unless she is new to the ward) already has a great deal of information about a number of the patients with whom she will be working. The only patients she will not know will be patients who have been admitted since she was last on duty.

▼ Because nurses already know most of the biographical details of the patients the report is kept very brief, concentrating only on matters that affect the patient's care in the next and subsequent shifts.

▼ Nurses are expected to consult the care plan for the details.

▼ Nurses receive a detailed report only on the patients with whom they are going to work, not for every patient on the ward.

▼ The main nurse delivering care to the patient on one shift hands over to the main nurse who will deliver care to her/him on the next.

CASE STUDY 1

COMMUNICATION AT HANDOVER:
Athlone Ward, Middlesex Hospital.

The method of allocation (primary nursing) already allowed nurses to work with the same patients throughout their length of stay. But Athlone Ward found it useful to use a couple of monthly staff meetings to review the conduct of the report and the value of the information passed from one shift to the next.

Nursing staff decided that it was not an effective use of time to receive details about all the patients on the ward at the start of the shift, as they had a communication board stating which patient was in bed at the entrance to the ward. A book was kept in the treatment room which provided details of any patient on the ward who was not to receive cardiopulmonary resuscitation. They agreed that every nurse was responsible for checking the book when arriving on duty.

They have found the system works well:

▼ it is a more effective use of time;

▼ it provides an opportunity for reciprocal communication between the patient and the nurses.

After first implementing the changes, they identified potential concerns:

▼ breach of confidentiality should other patients overhear;

▼ lack of opportunity for patients to 'opt out' should they wish;

▼ inexperienced nurses handing over inappropriate information.

These concerns have subsequently been overcome by the introduction of a nursing standard and further evaluation and research.

Communication between nurses and other health professions

82. Effective communication between nurses and professional colleagues from other disciplines, on and off the wards, requires agreement and understanding about how the channels of communication work and about roles and responsibilities. The need to keep open and discuss channels of communication is especially important in times of change.

83. The numbers of different people communicating with one another about the same patient needs to be kept to the minimum, and to include only those who are directly involved in the patient's care.

▼   The ward sister's role is to make explicit the correct channels of communication between nurses, doctors and the other health professionals involved with patients on her ward. She discusses and agrees in advance changes in customary practice affecting communication between nurses and others with everyone concerned, so that there can be no doubt in any one's mind about the communication system on the ward.

▼   She teaches junior members of nursing staff to communicate effectively with their professional colleagues. The teaching role extends to participating in meetings and attending ward rounds with students and juniors until they are competent to take full part in the process.

▼   She makes sure that multi-disciplinary meetings and case conferences happen, negotiating with medical staff and other professional colleagues to obtain their commitment to attend meetings.

▼   The nurse who attends these meetings is the nurse directly caring for the patient.

▼   The nurse who has the main responsibility for communicating with the patient is the main channel of communication on behalf of that patient with professional colleagues from other disciplines.

▼   The deputising arrangements for when she is not available are made in advance and are clearly understood.

(d) DISCHARGE PLANNING

84. The Department of Health's guidance on planning discharge from hospital is practical, comprehensive and a useful starting point (Ref.15). A number of hospitals and wards in the study sample were starting work to improve discharge planning. The emergent features in their work are:

▼ A hospital discharge policy that is clear, simple and practical. All members of staff are trained in implementing the policy, and a system is established for monitoring the policy, following-up samples of patients and collecting data on unplanned re-admissions.

▼ One nurse has overall responsibility for the discharge plan and for co-ordinating the discharge arrangements. This is the nurse who has the main responsibility for communicating with the patient and the relatives or carers.

▼ Every patient is assessed for discharge, although not all patients need an elaborate discharge plan. The assessment is completed at the initial patient assessment and history-taking, and the outcome is documented.

▼ At discharge, the patient is given written information to accompany the oral explanations about after-care, further appointments, drugs, self-care, and so on.

85. Although hospital managers and nursing staff will state the rules of good discharge planning ('preparation for discharge starts at admission'; 'the patient and the relatives/ carers must be consulted', and so on), generally speaking, the rules are still not being applied. The most likely explanation for the gap between the theory and actual practice lies in the fact that it is very difficult for hospital-based staff to hold on to an awareness of patients' lives outside hospital.

86. It may need a cultural shift in the awareness and attitudes of hospital-based staff for improvements to take place in discharge planning.

DISCHARGE PLANNING:
Christchurch Ward, Battle Hospital, Reading

Nurses on Christchurch Ward at Battle Hospital in Reading, succeeded in improving their discharge planning by using a quality improvement/ standard setting approach to implementing and evaluating change (see the first page of the discharge planning standard in Figure 3).

Before they set the standard, they recognised the need to do some research. Their objective was to achieve good discharge planning for a range of patient types, but they realised they knew very little about both their own discharge planning practice and what had happened to patients after they had been discharged and any problems they may have experienced.

They decided that some nurses should accompany discharged patients home, whilst others would conduct a short interview with previous patients on the telephone. The results of this relatively simple qualitative research exercise, together with systematic discussions about all the issues involved on the ward, brought about a profound change of awareness on the ward about the significance of hospital discharge to patients, and about their own practice.

For the first time, the meaning of continuity of care beyond the ward door came alive to them. They found it easier to visualise patients' home circumstances, became more interested in finding out about them, and understood the importance of assessing for discharge at the time of admission.

They take it in turns to rotate on standards monitoring duties for a period of months. The discharge planning standard is monitored continually (using the questionnaire in Figure 3, overleaf), and the results are fed back to the ward team at staff meetings. As problems come to light they are discussed, and action plans are drawn up to resolve them.

Figure 3: Page one of the standard

West Berkshire Health Authority

Standard Reference No...03.A.11.25...............

Topic...CONTINUITY OF CARE........................

Sub Topic...DISCHARGE PLANNING.......................

Application To...CHRISTCHURCH WARD...................

Achieve Standard By...MAY 1991.......................

Review Standard By...MAY 1992........................

Standard Compiled By...S/N S....../Sr B.............

Agreed By.................Director of Nursing Services

Standard Statement. Patients are not discharged from Christchurch Ward until arrangements for meeting their needs in the community have been completed.

© 1991

Structure	Process	Outcome
1. WBHA discharge policy and patient's nursing record and discharge plans are available. Nurses are given instruction on discharge planning orientation.	1. Preparation for patient's discharge begins on admission when nurses discuss: - social circumstances - known lifestyle - physical and mental capabilities - family support - existing social services support.	1. A comprehensive assessment of patient's home conditions is available.
2. Telephone/bleep numbers of health care professionals and referral sheets are available on the ward.	2. Nurses arrange early referral of patients requiring specialist assessment from occupational therapist/physiotherapist, and record of details in the patient's discharge plan and nursing records.	2. The patient has any specialist assessment completed before discharge.
3. Aircall system for contacting community personnel operates.	3. Nurses liaise and co-operate with health care professionals, community staff, social services and patient's relatives concerning: - home assessments - alterations to housing - equipment/aids required - home help and special support.	3. Necessary home alterations are completed before discharge, and any special equipment/aids to independence and social support are immediately available.

Structure	Process	Outcome
4. Self-medication sheets and DHSS patient information on social support are available on the ward.	4. Nurses discuss discharge arrangements with the patient and plan for and assist them with their individual needs in the community, including: - skill checks - self care - self medication - independence and mobility.	4. The patient is confident about their ability to cope at home.
5. Aircall and Response record from District Nurse is on the ward. Medication dispensed for patients to take home is delivered to the ward. Hospital care/fares assistance scheme is available for patients being discharged from hospital. Ambulance service is only to be used on medical grounds when established procedures followed. Ward diary is maintained and arrangements are made.	5. The patient's Primary Nurse is responsible for the safe co-ordination of patient's discharge home, and for ensuring the final arrangements are completed. Patients leave the hospital accompanied by a responsible person.	5. Patient's safety and continuity of care following discharge from hospital are assured.
6. Discharge letters are completed. Outpatients appointments made before patient discharge.	6. Before the patient leaves the ward the nurse ensures that patient, relatives, hospital and community personnel are fully informed and understand the discharge arrangements. Day Hospital referrals are confirmed. Relevant documentation is completed.	6. Misunderstandings and breakdowns in communication related to the patient's discharge and subsequent care at home do not occur.

Figure 3: Page two of the standard

Patients are not discharged from Christchurch Ward until arrangements for meeting
their needs in the community have been completed.

MONITORING PERIOD _____   WARD _____

MONITORING AGENT _____

MONITORING METHOD	CODE	CRITERIA	YES	NO	N/A	COMME
Records	1P & O	An assessment of patient's home circumstances is documented in nursing records				
Observe	1S	WBHA Discharge Policy is on the ward.				
Ask/observe	2P & O	Patients requiring specialist assessment receive this prior to discharge.				
Records	2P	Referral to Occupational Therapist/Physiotherapist is documented in nursing records				
Ask relatives	3P	Patient's relatives have discussed with ward staff the patient's home care needs.				
Ask Occupational Therapist and Social Worker	3O	- Any home alterations have been completed before discharge. - equipment aids are available for use on discharge. - Social support has been arranged to commence immediately after discharge.				
Ask nurses	4P	Nurse has discussed discharge plans with patient.				
Ask patient	4O	Patient feels able to cope at home.				
Observe	5S	Medication to be taken home by patient is delivered to ward.				
Observe/ask	5P & O	Primary nurse has completed and checked arrangements for patient discharge.				
Observe	5P	Patients are accompanied by a responsible person when discharged.				
Observe/ask	6S & P	Documentation pertaining to patient's discharge has been completed.				

Figure 3: Page three of the standard

CHRISTCHURCH WARD - BATTLE HOSPITAL

In order to help us to monitor our standard of discharge planning,
we would be grateful if you would complete this questionnaire with
reference to:

Hospital Label

Were the patient's care needs discussed with you over
the telephone prior to discharge?

Yes/No

Comments:

Was the nursing section completed on the discharge
letter?

Yes/No

Comments:

Were there any omissions?

Yes/No

Comments:

Are there any other comments that you wish to make about this patient's
discharge?

Thank you for your help.

Please return in the envelope provided, via internal mail, as soon as
possible.

ENHANCING PATIENT-CENTRED CARE
(e) PLANNING PATIENT CARE

87. The changes that have been outlined, especially those affecting methods of patient-nurse allocation and rules of clinical decision-making, provide the context that has potential to motivate nurses to document individualised plans of care. In addition:

▼ The relevance of documenting care plans to the delivery of personalised care is underlined in the ward philosophy or statement of values.

▼ The ward sister and managers actively demonstrate the value they attach to care planning by showing an interest in completed care plans, and expecting nurses to refer to records at report and in teaching sessions.

▼ The time it takes to plan care properly is explicitly acknowledged.

▼ Care plans and continuation sheets are clearly signed and dated.

▼ Nurses complete care plans and records during the shift, as much as possible by the patient's bedside. The documentation is not left to the end of the shift, it is not delegated to someone who does not know the patient, and it is not done at home.

▼ Nurses rely on the plans for information about the patients. They refer to them at handover and during the shift, and they direct new and temporary members of staff to them for information about patients.

▼ The plans include enough detailed information for any nurse involved with the patient to be able to find out everything she needs to know both about the patient's clinical condition and personal preferences.

▼ If the ward uses standardised or core care plans, they are individualised. Where care planning has been computerised, there is scope for free text to allow the plan to be adapted to the person.

(f) THE PATIENT'S DAY

88. The patient is consulted over how s/he likes to spend the day and the timing of events (e.g. when s/he will wake up, wash, rest, have visitors).

▼　The patient's preferences are documented in the care plan. Within the limits of what is clinically permissible and practicable for the ward, the patient's preferences determine the shape of the day.

▼　The nurse responsible for the clinical decisions affecting the patient's care will discuss the plan of care with the medical staff and establish the clinical requirements governing the timing of treatment for that individual patient.

6

Managing For Quality

INTRODUCTION

89. The purpose of this final section of the handbook is to show by practical example how sisters and managers can not only cope with change, but become successful leaders of the change process.

90. The health service is full of talk about 'quality' and 'the management of change', but how do managers and ward sisters with new responsibilities know where to start? One of the best ways is to see what other people are doing, to visit other wards and hospitals and talk to the people involved. The section ends with a list of contact names and addresses of people that may be useful.

91. If it is not possible to visit other wards and hospitals, reading about what other people are doing is, perhaps, the next best option. The concluding section of the handbook is therefore organised around two case studies. The first, shows how the general principles of quality assurance have been introduced at Battle Hospital in Reading. The work that nurses and managers are doing in the hospital demonstrates that, provided one goes about it in the right way, it is possible to achieve measurable improvements in the quality of patient care. The final case study, brings the rhetoric of 'change-management' to life. It tells the story of how a Clinical Nurse Manager (CNM) and a team of sisters changed the organisation of care within a clinical area.

QUALITY ASSURANCE

92. The general principles of successful quality improvement programmes are well-established. They are about finding the right balance between leadership at the top and autonomy at the bottom; between the senior managers' commitment to quality assurance and the freedom for groups of staff to look at their practice and make their own decisions about how to improve it. Improving quality is a con-

tinuous process that comes about through practitioners acquiring tools and techniques to examine what they are doing. The essential tools are skills in setting standards, monitoring and action planning.

93. The RCN's DySSSy system (Ref. 16) has done a great deal to develop and demonstrate the application of general principles to quality improvements within nursing. This is partly through the work it has done on refining the methodology for monitoring standards, and through the various activities and organisations associated with it: e.g. facilitation and group skills workshops, and the Quality Assurance Network. The latter publishes a newsletter, and holds meetings and conferences.

94. The work described in Case Study 3 puts the principles into practice. It takes two starting points for granted. An assumption that it is always possible to make changes for the better, no matter how intractable the situation. Everyone wants to do good work, and nurses are basically motivated by the desire to help people. And the assumption that it is best to begin with whatever material presents itself as relevant to *this* area of work, and *this* group of staff, at *this* particular time.

CASE STUDY 3

SETTING STANDARDS
Battle Hospital, Reading

One of the organisational pre-requisites for standard setting (or any quality improvement) is a forum that brings staff (including night staff) together. At Battle, where shift overlaps last less than an hour, staff meetings on wards usually take place in the late afternoon or early evening.

The standard setting process on a ward begins with a group discussion – led by the Senior Practice Development Nurse who has had training in group work and facilitation – about, in very general terms, how staff 'would like things to be'. The Practice Development Nurse describes this process as '*like putting a mirror up to the nurses that allows them to see what they are doing.*'

Gradually, the conclusions from the general discussion about what staff would like the ward to be like are condensed down into short statements that can be written down. The statements spell out the philosophy of the ward and the values of the team, and from there staff begin to explore what they mean in practical terms. Which areas of their work, and what happens on the ward in particular, express their values? And what do they need to change to bring their practice in to line with their aspirations?

The length of time the process takes varies in different parts of the hospital depending on a number of factors. These include: the nature of the clinical work, the dynamics of the group, and staff morale. In some cases staff have written the philosophy themselves after two meetings; in others, it has taken twice weekly meetings over a period of a month or more with the Practice Development Nurse acting as facilitator and helping them to write the philosophy.

Once the group has succeeded in identifying a specific area of practice they want to develop, they begin the process of standard setting. There is no single right way of going about this. Sometimes it involves members of the nursing team in a short period of study and research; sometimes it emerges out of group discussions that look at the detail of how the ward works.

At this stage of the process the key is to set a standard that is achievable and that can be measured, and to agree a method for monitoring it. (Appendix 1 shows two of the standards developed out of this process on two acute general wards.) Once a standard has been set and is being monitored, the results of the monitoring are fed back to the group of staff. (See Appendix 1 for examples of monitoring methods.)

At Battle, the monitoring is usually done by a group of three to four nurses from any/every grade. The monitoring nurses are either elected by the ward team or they volunteer for the job. They serve on the monitoring team for periods of up to six months. Monitoring involves them in some additional work, but as far as possible they include it in their normal way of working. They do it continually, usually monthly, and it can involve observation, interviewing patients and their visitors, or checking nursing records. The results of their work are discussed at staff meetings, and where there is a need to take action – either to stop the standard falling, or, if the standard is being met, to develop it further – the staff group develops an action plan.

GENERAL LESSONS IN THE MANAGEMENT OF WARD-BASED NURSING
THE ROLE OF THE WARD SISTER

95. The ward sister holds the key to the ward: her management style determines the ethos and direction of the ward and its response to change.

96. The sisters managing the more patient-centred wards in the study sample are not all the same age, they trained at different times and they are at different stages in their careers. But they do have two things in common: they see their role clearly, and they have enough authority and autonomy to bring about improvements in patient care.

97. They do not necessarily all have the same view of the sister's role – some put more emphasis on clinical work, others on facilitating and developing staff. But

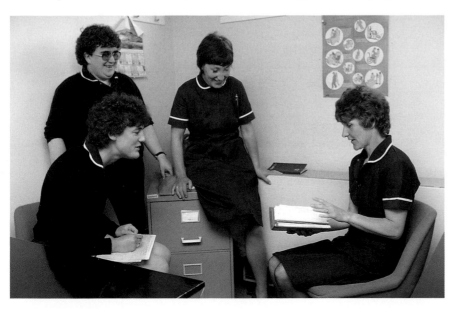

they all see skills in planning, delegation, negotiation and communication as the most important.

> **SISTER A:** *'I am the co-ordinator and the facilitator of everything the staff do on the ward. I don't do everything myself, but I do know everything that goes on. As much as possible, I like to get the staff involved in doing some of the more 'traditional' elements of the sister's role. That's why we started a system of self assessment in pairs, so that they do not come to me for everything.'*

> **SISTER B:** *'I think my role is to think ahead and plan what will happen on the ward, and also to be the clinical leader. To do that I need to be a bit removed. I need to take time away so that I'm not always just reacting to the latest crisis, and so I've had to spend alot of time with my F grade deputy working out our separate roles.'*

> **SISTER C:** *'I have to be included on the off-duty, and I don't have as much time as I would like to develop the ward. But I work very closely with the junior sister, and we have learned to delegate an awful lot of the work I used to do to the others. Each team does its own roster now and the junior sister checks it and makes sure of the cover for the whole ward. The other thing is we've got better at having systems. Systems for ordering so that the ward clerk can do it, for induction and for students' training. We've found it saves time in the long run.'*

98. Innovative sisters succeed in improving patient care through a combination of their own individual qualities and skills and the character of the management environment in which they operate (Box C).

THE WARD SISTER'S MANAGER

99. Regardless of whether their background is in nursing or general management, the effective managers at this level also have a clear understanding of what can be achieved, and ground themselves firmly in knowing what is happening on the wards, clinically and as well as in other respects.

100. Their knowledge derives partly from direct, personal contact with patients and staff, but also from collecting, or causing other departments (personnel, finance, planning and information, quality etc.) to collect systematic data. They use the information at their disposal both to compare different wards, and to

monitor developments on the same ward over time. It is a useful tool in helping sisters on wards that lag behind set objectives and in sharing the good practice of the more advanced wards across all the wards in their span of control.

101. They conduct their relationship to the wards through the ward sister but they do not interfere with either her management of the ward or her relationship with her staff. Instead, they consult and involve her in decisions about the ward's resources, and actively involve themselves in agreeing with the sister the framework of objectives and standards within which she will manage.

102. On staff development, for example, one manager agreed a programme for staff development with the ward sisters in her Clinical Directorate. The programme identifies the skills and qualifications required for every post and grade and for every individual member of staff within the first two years of appointment.

103. The programme provides the framework within which sisters agree 'learning contracts' with their staff, and plan training and study leave for up to a year ahead. In this way, sisters are directly involved in staff development, and can make sure that the staff member's learning contract combines her own professional aspirations with the training needs of the Directorate or Unit.

104. One of the key functions of managers outside the wards is to negotiate with medical consultants and other managers the parameters of workload, staffing, quality and budgets within which the nursing service is provided. It is more efficient to negotiate on behalf of a group of wards than a single ward and where managers take on this role, it leaves ward sisters free to get on with the business of running their ward.

CASE STUDY 4

CHANGING THE ORGANISATION OF CARE:
Renal Services, Hope Hospital, Salford

The case study begins with the Clinical Nurse Manager (CNM) of Renal Services at Hope Hospital, now Senior Nurse Manager for the Clinical Directorate of Medicine.

Her understanding of her role was that she was the patient's advocate; she saw her main task as being continuously to improve standards of care; her route into it, through valuing the nursing staff.

She was quite clear in her own mind that there is a difference between leadership and taking a top-down approach to quality improvement. She saw it as essential that she should know the clinical areas and have an analysis of their various philosophies, strengths and weaknesses. But against that background, her task was not to take the clinical areas over, to set standards for them, or to lead the teams in setting them. It was to meet the sisters and plan a strategy with them for improving quality.

In the meetings with sisters, she set out what she expected, asked them what they were doing and then left it to them to work out how they were going to achieve the objectives. She always made clear that they could come back to her for help, advice or guidance and that she would seek additional help for them if it was needed. She provided them with references for good practice and professional guidelines wherever possible.

When she was identifying her own objectives, the CNM envisaged that the introduction of primary nursing was achievable by the end of the first year within the Renal Services.

Each of the clinical areas had previously had its own particular way of organising care, although all of them saw themselves as doing individualised nursing care. The sisters had relatively little contact with each other's areas, but all of them faced similar difficulties and problems. The Nurse Manager acknowledged that the sisters needed to discuss collectively their understanding of their own role and general issues in management.

She presented six factors to the sisters which, when addressed would provide the foundations for change. They needed to:

▼ Develop management competencies for the sisters to enable them to become the professional and managerial leader of their clinical area, and to nurture and ensure the quality of their teams. (They could use the existing staff appraisal system to do this.)

▼ Create a climate for change.

▼ Empower nursing staff below F grade to be autonomous within the bounds of their own professional knowledge and clinical skills.

▼ Develop nurses' confidence in decision-making, inter-personal and organisational skills, so that they could form the necessary relationships with patients, carers and multi-disciplinary teams.

▼ Explain the organisation and management of nursing care to the medical staff and other professional colleagues.

▼ Tell patients, carers and visitors to the areas what they were doing.

She asked the nine sisters to write short papers identifying the pros and cons of changing to primary nursing. The sisters were to consider the changes that would need to be made in their own area down to the last detail. Where these were likely to entail major changes in rosters, shifts and mentoring systems, they were to include in their papers worked examples of how to overcome the problems.

During a six week period, although they were free to return to the manager at any time for help, the sisters spent the time talking to their staff about the issues and getting them involved in thinking through the potential problems.

The CNM wrote a summary of the nine papers and presented the results at a further meeting. Together they discussed outstanding problems, agreed a timetable and set a date for reviewing their progress towards primary nursing. They also agreed on a strategy for monitoring the changes and a means to feed back the results through further meetings.

The approach empowered the sisters to take responsibility for the re-organisation of patient care within their areas. And it also allowed all the staff to contribute their views to the framework for change and have ownership of the process.

References

1. Audit Commission (1991) *The Virtue of Patients: Making Best Use of Ward Nursing Resources.* HMSO, London

2. B. Moores and A.G.H. Thompson (1986) What 1357 hospital inpatients think about aspects of their stay in British acute hospitals. *Journal of Advanced Nursing*, 11, 87-102

3. B. Friend (1992) Record recovery. *Nursing Times*, 88, No.2, pp. 34-35

4. R. Waite, J. Buchan and J. Thomas (1989) *Nurses In and Out of Work.* IMS Report No. 170: Institute of Manpower Studies: Falmer, Brighton

5. Mersey Regional Health Authority Department of Nursing (1989) *Job Satisfaction. A Survey of Nurses, Midwives and Health Visitors: their attitude towards, and satisfaction with, work in Mersey Region.*

6. Price Waterhouse (1988) *Nurse Retention and Recruitment: a matter of priority.* London

7. D. Thompson (1989) Management of the Patient with Acute Myocardial Infarction. *Nursing Standard*, 4, pp. 34-38

8. D. Thompson (1988) Sources and patterns of anxiety in coronary patients. *Nursing Times*, 84, p. 58

9. Royal College of Surgeons, College of Anaesthetists (1990) *Report of the Working Party on Pain after Surgery*, London

10. V. Henderson (1966) *The Nature of Nursing: A Definition and its Implications for Practice, Research and Education.* New York: Macmillan

11. S. G. Wright (1986) *Building and Using a Model of Nursing.* London: Edward Arnold

12. Department of Health Nursing Division (1989) *Strategy for Nursing.* HMSO, London

13. *The Patients' Charter* (1991) HMSO, London

14. Audit Commission (1992) *Lying in Wait: The Use of Medical Beds in Acute Hospitals*. HMSO, London

15. Department of Health (1989) *Discharge of Patients from Hospital*. DoH Circular HC/89/5

16. A. Kitson (1990) *Quality Patient Care: An Introduction to the Dynamic Standard Setting System*. RCN: Scutari, London